A. FILEVSKI

The Only Food Supplement Book You'll Ever Need

A Complete Guide to Weight Loss, Muscle Growth, and Overall Health Enhancement

Contents

1

Introduction

This book dives into the science behind popular food supplements such as protein powders, creatine, branched-chain amino acids (BCAAs), and more. It explores how these supplements work at the molecular level, their proven health benefits, and the myths surrounding them. Chapters discuss the role of protein in muscle repair and growth, how creatine enhances strength and performance, and the thermogenic effects of certain fat-burning supplements. The book also includes practical advice on dosages, safety, and how to integrate supplements with a balanced diet to achieve weight loss or muscle gain goals.

The topic of this book is important because it addresses the growing interest in optimizing health and fitness through nutrition and supplementation, a trend that aligns with the increasing focus on active lifestyles and personal well-being. **You** should care because supplements like protein, creatine, and others can significantly impact physical performance, recovery, and overall health when used correctly. Whether aiming to lose weight, build muscle, or simply maintain a healthy body, supplements can play a role in complementing diet and exercise. Nowadays the market hype around protein powder, creatine, pre-workout and other food supplements can lead **You** to buy useless products that won't benefit your well-being at all. It will only hurt your pocket.

I strongly believe **You** should read this book because it provides a clear, evidence-based guide to understanding food supplements and their impact on health and fitness.

My name is Alexander. I'm a med student. I've been working out for 8 years now and learned a lot of things throughout my fitness journey. I'm a person that supports an active lifestyle and people who want to change for the better, whether that be people who want to lose weight, gain muscle or just want to be happy when they look at themselves in the mirror. In addition, I am writing this book because I want to end the misconception surrounding food supplements once and for all.

2

Protein Powder

What Is Protein Powder?

Protein powder is a nutritional supplement that can play a role in gaining muscle, losing weight and can help repair tissue. But, what really is protein powder? It essentially is protein mixed with other amino acids, carbohydrates and sweeteners.

Protein is the most important macro molecule in our organism. Our muscles, hair, eyes, organs, and many hormones and enzymes are primarily made out of protein. Each molecule of protein is basically made out of 20 amino acids. We can create 11 of the 20 amino acids. The other 9 are called essential amino acids. To fully understand the meaning of protein we need to understand how our bodies absorb protein and how we build muscle tissue from it.

First and foremost, when we consume any type of food, our enzymes break down bigger molecules (or macromolecules) such as proteins, carbs, and fats into smaller molecules(

micromolecules). Protein digestion begins when we start chewing the food in our mouth. Enzymes such as amylase and lipase start breaking down carbs and fats. Once the food reaches our stomach hydrochloric acid and enzymes called proteases break it down into smaller chains of amino acids. In your stomach, smaller amino acid chains travel to your small intestine. Meanwhile, your pancreas releases enzymes and a bicarbonate buffer to neutralize the acidity of the digested food. This neutralization enables additional enzymes to further break down the chains into individual amino acids. Protein absorption occurs in the small intestine, where tiny, finger-like structures called microvilli enhance the surface area for nutrient absorption. This maximizes the uptake of amino acids and other nutrients. After absorption, amino acids enter the bloodstream, which transports them to cells throughout the body to aid in tissue repair and muscle building.

Now that we know what protein powder, protein and protein absorption are we can move on to…

What are the benefits of Protein Powder?

All protein powders provide a very convenient source of high quality protein. If you are a person that doesn't have time to prepare meals immediately after a workout or simply isn't able to consume foods that are rich in protein every single day, then protein powder is the way to go. Every protein shake also contains essential amino acids, especially leucine, which is vital for muscle protein synthesis.

Protein powder helps repair and rebuild muscles after exercise, making it ideal for people engaging in strength training.

Another upside to protein powder consumption is that when you consume it, it will make you feel fuller for a longer period of time. That will result in eating less snacks which will make you maintain your desired weight or even lose weight as well.

Taking whey protein before a meal can trigger insulin release, which helps transport glucose into cells for energy or storage. As a result, post-meal blood sugar levels may decrease. However, the impact of protein on blood sugar regulation differs among individuals, influenced by factors such as the quantity and timing of protein consumption, as well as individual metabolic responses.

What are the negatives of Protein Powder?

Since protein powder is a dietary supplement the FDA leaves it up to the manufacturers to evaluate the safety of it. Therefore, we can't be 100% certain that a protein powder contains what the manufacturer says it contains.

The long term effects are also unknown due to the fact that there is limited information about the possible side effects of protein powder consumption in the long run.

Earlier this year, the Clean Label Project, a nonprofit organization, published a report highlighting the presence of toxins in protein powders. Researchers tested 134 products for 130 different toxins and discovered that many contained harmful substances, including heavy metals like lead, arsenic, cadmium, and mercury, as well as bisphenol-A (BPA, a chemical used in plastics), pesticides, and other contaminants linked to cancer and various health issues. In some cases, the toxin levels were alarmingly high; one protein powder, for instance, had 25 times the permitted amount of BPA.

Types of Protein Powder

There are many types of protein powders such as whey, casein, soy, pea and hemp.

I'm going to give you a short summary of all the types of whey proteins since they are the most accessible type of protein powder.

Whey proteins

Whey proteins are the most famous type of protein powder around. It is a mixture of proteins isolated from whey, the liquid material created as a by-product of cheese production. It contains all of the amino acids that our body needs. Whey is absorbed quickly making it an excellent choice for a post workout meal. There are three main types of whey proteins on the market: whey isolate, whey hydro-isolate and whey concentrate.

Hydro-isolate

Hydro-isolate whey protein uses a process called hydrolysis which partially digests whey protein isolate using enzymes, breaking longer amino acid chains into shorter peptides. This process creates "whey protein peptides," also called hydrolyzed whey or whey protein hydrolysate. The supposed benefits include improved digestion, especially for those sensitive to lactose, and faster absorption due to the smaller peptide size, though research is inconclusive.

Whey protein isolate

Whey protein isolate undergoes more processing than concentrate, which makes it more expensive ,but higher in protein, with minimal lactose and fat. This form is ideal for post-workout recovery and is commonly used in studies comparing whey to other protein sources.

Whey protein concentrate

Whey protein concentrate is the least processed whey protein option available on the market which makes it the cheapest option. It typically contains around 80% protein, 3.5% lactose, and 7.2% fat. If you're looking to spend as little money as possible on protein powder this is your choice.

Consumption

Protein Powder shouldn't be your primary source of protein. Having a balanced diet, sufficient water consumption, an active and healthy lifestyle all play a major role in a safe consumption of protein powder. The main idea of protein powder is to add 30-40 grams of protein to your daily protein intake if you're looking to gain muscle or lose fat. The daily recommended use is 1 scoop of protein powder (this can vary depending on your protein powder) mixed with 300 ml of water or milk. I believe you should only consume protein powder after a workout and take a break from it every once in a while.

take a break from it every once in a while.

3

Creatine

What is creatine?

Creatine is a naturally occurring compound found primarily in muscle cells. It plays a major role in energy production, especially during high-intensity physical activities like weightlifting, sprinting, and other short-duration exercises. Our bodies naturally produce a small amount of creatine. It is synthesized in our liver, kidneys and pancreas from amino acids.

Its main purpose is to create energy that is used by our muscles to contract. Creatine is stored in our muscle cells in the form of phosphocreatine and is used quickly to regenerate Adenosine triphosphate, which is the primary source of energy of all living organisms. Creatine is found in red meat, fish, chicken and even grape juice. The main problem is that in order to acquire your daily dose of creatine which typically is 5 grams, you would need to eat 2 pounds of steak (0,91 KG) every single day. That is the main reason why so many people buy pure creatine in the form of powder, capsules and others.

What are the benefits of creatine?

Let's take a deep dive into all the benefits of creatine. To start, creatine is suitable for all types of athletes. With creatine, muscles can perform at higher intensities for a longer duration, which can lead to better training sessions and overall progress. Creatine supplementation often results in noticeable gains in muscle size. This is partly due to an increase in water retention in muscle cells and partly due to enhanced workout performance. There is a chance that you'll gain 33% more muscle during your first few months of supplementing with creatine, 25% more muscle during your first year, and 15% more muscle during your first decade but that is mainly determined by your genetics. By promoting cell hydration and creating an anabolic environment, creatine supports the processes necessary for muscle repair and growth which is a key factor in building additional muscle mass.

Creatine also has some cognitive benefits. Just like muscles, the brain relies on ATP for energy. Creatine supplementation can enhance brain energy metabolism, especially under demanding conditions like sleep deprivation or mental fatigue. Some studies suggest creatine may improve short-term memory, reaction time, and cognitive performance, particularly in vegetarians and older adults who may have lower baseline levels. Preliminary research hints at the potential for creatine to support brain health, reducing the risk of neurodegenerative diseases like Parkinson's or Alzheimer's, though more studies are needed.

As I said, many swimmers, tennis players, soccer players and other athletes use creatine. These athletes engage in activities that demand a combination of explosive power, sustained effort, and quick recovery, all of which creatine supports effectively.

Studies note a rise in hormones, such as IGF-1, after taking creatine. IGF-1. Insulin-like growth factor 1 is a hormone that has a similar structure to insulin. It plays an important role in childhood growth, and has anabolic effects in adults.

Research also indicates that creatine may lower blood sugar levels and help treat nonalcoholic fatty liver disease. However, more research in these areas is needed.

What are the negatives of creatine?

Creatine increases the water content in muscle cells, leading to water retention. This can result in gaining 2-6 lbs (1-3 kg) of additional weight. This can be a problem for athletes in specific weight classes or activities requiring agility. The good thing is that most of this weight is water and not fat and with time it will stabilize.

Taking too much creatine at once or consuming it on an empty stomach can irritate the digestive system. Some of the symptoms may be diarrhea, bloating or cramping. You can manage this by splitting your dose into smaller doses throughout the day, mixed with a little more water.

Creatine draws water into muscle cells, which can reduce water availability for other parts of the body. This can result in dehydration. The smartest way to avoid this is to drink plenty of water (2,5 - 3 litres a day).

A 2009 study suggested a connection between creatine supplements and increased levels of DHT, a hormone associated with hair loss. However, the majority of research does not support this correlation.

Different types of creatine

Creatine monohydrate

Creatine monohydrate is the most famous and best type of creatine. This form of creatine has been used in the majority of research on the topic. This means that all the benefits that creatine provides have been observed almost exclusively when creatine monohydrate was used.

This form is made up of a creatine molecule and a water molecule. By removing the water molecule, creatine anhydrous is created which has less concentration of water and more creatine. Theoretically creatine anhydrous is better than monohydrate simply because it has more creatine molecules right? Well, no. Although there are slight differences in processing, all these forms are likely equally effective when taken in equal doses.

Creatine monohydrate is one of the most studied and effective supplements on the market, with a strong safety profile when used as directed. Creatine monohydrate has been the benchmark for this supplement due to its safety, effectiveness, and affordability.

Creatine Ethyl Ester

Creatine ethyl ester (CEE) is a modified form of creatine where a molecule of ethanol is attached to the creatine molecule. This modification is intended to enhance its absorption and bioavailability compared to creatine monohydrate. Some people claim that creatine ethyl ester may result in better muscle uptake and require smaller doses to achieve the same effects. However, research has generally found that creatine monohydrate is equally or more effective, with no consistent evidence that CEE provides superior benefits. As a result, CEE is less commonly used than creatine monohydrate.

Creatine Hydrochloride

Creatine hydrochloride (HCl) has become increasingly popular among manufacturers and supplement users, likely due to claims of its enhanced solubility.

Its higher solubility in water has led to speculation that lower doses might be effective, potentially reducing common side effects like stomach upset. However, this remains unproven until tested.

One study reported that creatine HCl is 38 times more soluble than creatine monohydrate. Despite this, there are no published studies on the effects of creatine HCl in humans.

Given the extensive evidence supporting creatine monohydrate, creatine HCl cannot be considered superior until direct comparisons are made through research.

Creatine Magnesium Chelate

Creatine magnesium chelate is a type of creatine where magnesium is chemically bonded to the creatine molecule.

A study compared the effects of creatine monohydrate, creatine magnesium chelate, and a placebo on bench press strength and endurance. Both creatine forms outperformed the placebo, but there was no significant difference between the two.

This suggests that while creatine magnesium chelate may be an effective option, it does not appear to offer advantages over standard creatine monohydrate.

Consumption

Many people begin creatine supplementation with a loading phase to quickly increase muscle creatine levels.

To follow a loading phase, consume 20 grams of creatine per day for 5–7 days, dividing this into four 5-gram servings throughout the day. Taking it with a carb- or protein-rich meal may enhance absorption.

After the loading phase, a daily maintenance dose of 3–5 grams is sufficient to keep muscle creatine levels elevated. Since cycling creatine offers no additional benefits, this dosage can be maintained long-term.

If you prefer to skip the loading phase, simply take 3–5 grams per day, but it may take about four weeks to fully saturate your muscle stores.

Because creatine draws water into muscle cells, it's important to take it with a glass of water and stay hydrated throughout the day.

4

Pre-Workout

What is pre-workout?

Pre-workouts are food supplements designed to boost your energy and athletic performance. These are usually powdered supplements that are mixed with water and consumed before a workout.

Nitric oxide is a naturally occurring compound in the body that helps relax blood vessels and enhance blood flow. Pre-workout supplements often contain ingredients that support nitric oxide production, such as L-arginine, L-citrulline, and dietary nitrate sources like beetroot juice.

Besides giving you energy, pre-workouts enhance your focus, increase your overall endurance, increase your strength and pump.

The 5 most important ingredients you should look for when buying pre-workout are: L-Citrulline; Caffeine; Creatine; Beta Alanine and Electrolytes. Those five ingredients cover all of the boxes I mentioned above.

What are the benefits of pre-workout?

What if I tell you that there is a magical pill that *will* turn the most tired, the most demotivated, the most crappy day into a perfect day for a workout. Well that magical pill is pre-workout. Besides the positives I listed above there are other benefits I haven't mentioned yet.

Certain ingredients in pre-workouts may help reduce muscle soreness and improve post-workout recovery, enabling quicker turnaround times between training sessions.

Some pre-workout formulas contain thermogenic ingredients (e.g., caffeine, green tea extract) that may help increase calorie burn and support fat loss.

Beta-alanine can help buffer acid buildup in muscles, reducing the burn associated with intense exercise and potentially allowing for longer or more intense workouts.

What are the negatives of pre-workout?

Pre-workout supplements often contain artificial sweeteners or sugar alcohols.These ingredients improve flavor without adding calories, but some sweeteners can cause digestive issues.In particular, consuming large amounts of sugar alcohols may lead to symptoms like gas, bloating, and diarrhea, which can interfere with your workout.Some individuals also experience similar digestive discomfort from certain artificial sweeteners, such as sucralose, though these effects have not been scientifically confirmed.It may be best to avoid pre-workouts with high levels of these sweeteners, or start with a small dose to gauge your tolerance.

Caffeine is the primary energy-boosting ingredient in most

pre-workout supplements.Consuming too much caffeine can lead to side effects like elevated blood pressure, poor sleep, and increased stress.Most pre-workout servings contain roughly the same amount of caffeine as 1–2 cups (240–475 mL) of coffee. However, if you consume caffeine from other sources during the day, you might unintentionally exceed a safe amount.

Consumption

Most pre-workout supplements come with instructions on how to use them.

While it's important to follow these guidelines, it's also a good idea to start with a smaller dose to test your tolerance, especially if the product contains caffeine or beta-alanine.

If the supplement includes beta-alanine, don't be alarmed if you experience a tingling sensation; it's harmless, though some people may find it uncomfortable.

Pre-workouts are typically taken 30–60 minutes before exercising to allow the ingredients time to enter your bloodstream and take effect.

Lastly, if your pre-workout contains caffeine or other stimulants, consider the timing of your intake to avoid interfering with your sleep.

Do not exceed the recommended dosage!

5

Amino Acids

What are amino acids?

Amino acids are vital compounds that play numerous crucial roles in the body, such as synthesizing neurotransmitters and hormones, forming proteins, digesting food, repairing tissues, and providing energy.

Often called the building blocks of life, the human body requires 20 different amino acids to perform all its functions.

Amino acids are categorized into three main types: essential amino acids, nonessential amino acids, and conditionally essential amino acids.

In this chapter I will talk about both Essential Amino Acid and Branched-chain amino acids and compare them.

What are ESSENTIAL AMINO ACIDS

Nine of the 20 amino acids essential for the body's functions are classified as essential amino acids (EAAs). These cannot be produced by the body, so they must be obtained through your diet.

Without these EAAs, the body cannot function optimally. The nine EAAs are histidine, leucine, methionine, threonine, valine, isoleucine, lysine, phenylalanine, and tryptophan.

BCAAs are a specific group of essential amino acids (EAAs), meaning that when you consume EAAs, you're also benefiting from the effects of BCAAs.

What are BRANCHED-CHAIN AMINO ACIDS?

Branched-chain amino acids (BCAAs) are a subset of essential amino acids (EAAs). This means that while all BCAAs are EAAs, not all EAAs are BCAAs.

The term "branched chain" refers to the structure of the molecules that make up BCAAs.

Three of the nine EAAs are considered BCAAs, including leucine, isoleucine, and valine.

Leucine is essential for your body to produce protein and repair muscles after intense exercise. It also plays a key role in synthesizing growth hormones, maintaining healthy blood sugar levels, and aiding in recovery from injuries. Leucine is commonly found in foods like fish, poultry, meat, eggs, and milk.

Isoleucine is a branched-chain amino acid (BCAA) stored in muscle tissue. The body uses isoleucine to build new muscle tissue, maintain energy levels, support immune function, and produce hemoglobin.

Valine is an amino acid that helps support healthy energy levels, promotes muscle repair and recovery, and stimulates muscle growth. It is most commonly found in foods such as meat, soy, fish, and dairy.

Main Differences

BCAAs gained popularity primarily because of their specific role in muscle metabolism and their high concentration in muscle tissue. They were marketed as a targeted solution for muscle recovery and growth, and the simplicity of a supplement containing just three amino acids made them especially appealing. The fitness industry also embraced BCAAs for their versatility—they were easy to mix with water or a workout shake, tasted pleasant, and were more affordable than full EAA supplements. For individuals focused on weight loss or fasting, BCAAs were seen as a way to preserve muscle mass without the added calories from whole proteins.

As our understanding of muscle physiology has advanced, it's become clear that while BCAAs are important, they aren't the entire picture. The growing popularity of EAAs in the supplement world reflects a deeper understanding of muscle growth. To optimize muscle protein synthesis, the body requires all the building blocks found in the full spectrum of EAAs, not just the three present in BCAAs.

In summary, while BCAAs can aid in muscle recovery and remain useful in specific situations like fasting or low-calorie diets, EAAs provide a more complete and effective solution for muscle building. The shift from BCAAs to EAAs is based on a more thorough approach to muscle protein synthesis.

For those serious about maximizing gains, EAAs are the superior choice. They supply everything your muscles need to grow, repair, and perform at their peak, making them the preferred option for athletes and fitness enthusiasts.

Consumption

It's recommended to take EAAs or BCAAs either during, right before, or immediately after an intense workout. This timing may help reduce muscle soreness and enhance your anabolic rate, promoting faster muscle growth.

6

Mass Gainers

What are mass gainers?

Mass gainers are supplements that combine carbs, protein, and fats, designed to help you gain weight, particularly if you're aiming to bulk up. They can be a useful source of additional calories and protein, especially when you're looking to build muscle during intense training periods. Mass gainers typically have a carb-to-protein ratio of either 3:1 or 2:1. Some formulas also include micronutrients, such as vitamins and minerals, in varying quantities.

Many mass gainers provide up to three times more calories per serving than regular protein powders. While the increased calorie count is the main factor behind the effectiveness of these products, more isn't always better—there's a fine line between maintaining weight and gaining it.

What are the benefits of mass gainers?

If you find it difficult to meet your daily calorie goals due to financial or time constraints but still want to ensure you're eating enough to make progress in the gym or with your weight goals, a mass gainer could be a helpful solution.

It's also important to address the "hardgainer" stereotype—the idea that some people have an unusually high metabolism and don't respond as expected to moderate increases in calorie intake. While this idea is debated, it does have some support in scientific literature. Greg Nuckols, M.A. in Sport Science and editor of the *MASS Research Review*, shared his perspective on the issue:

"When people go into caloric surpluses, the body tries to stay close to maintenance by compensating. There may be small increases in metabolic rate, but the larger compensations tend to happen through increases in non-exercise activity thermogenesis (NEAT). Some individuals experience minor increases in NEAT during a caloric surplus, while others may see significant increases. These compensatory changes in NEAT could make it more challenging to achieve a substantial caloric surplus, especially if you don't have a large appetite."

What are the negatives of mass gainers?

Mass gainers won't add lean muscle mass on its own. If you take the marketing at face value, you're likely to be disappointed. Mass gainers are simply a high-calorie source of protein and carbohydrates, not a miracle solution.

Additionally, the ingredients in most common mass gainers raise some concerns for certain populations. A significant portion of the calorie content typically comes from maltodextrin and other additives, which may be a dealbreaker for individuals with diabetes or those trying to avoid high Glycemic Index (GI) sugars. Mass gainers are also generally not compatible with a ketogenic diet, which focuses on high-protein, high-fat macros while avoiding carbs.

Common additives like egg, soy, and whey protein may pose issues for those who are lactose intolerant. Moreover, many mass gainers contain relatively high-fat content, which can slow protein absorption and may not be ideal when consumed immediately after a workout.

Upset stomach: Mass gainers can cause digestive issues for individuals with food intolerances. If you're trying a mass gainer for the first time, it's a good idea to start with a smaller dose and gradually increase it. It's common to experience flatulence, bloating, and cramps during the first week of use.

Consumption

Mass gainer can also be consumed in the morning before breakfast, when the stomach is still empty. After 6-8 hours of fasting overnight, your body is in a near-fasting state, and many cells aren't getting the nutrients they need.

Drinking a mass gainer shake for breakfast is beneficial because your body can fully utilize the nutrients without interference from other foods. The calories, protein, carbs, vitamins, and minerals provide essential fuel for your body and muscles.

It also helps kickstart your metabolism in the morning, even before you get out of bed. These calories can activate your metabolic rate, putting your body into an anabolic muscle-building state to begin the day.

Another ideal time to take a mass gainer is 30 minutes to an hour before your workout. This is when your body can effectively use the calories and nutrients for energy, strength, endurance, and focus during your gym session.

Another great time to take a mass gainer is within 30 to 60 minutes after your workout. At this point, your muscles are likely depleted of glycogen—the stored carbohydrate your body uses for energy—and may even be slightly damaged from intense training.

In my humble opinion mass gainers are unnecessary. They can help a person gain weight but eating one or two more meals a day will always be superior.

7

Fat Burners

What are fat burners?

Fat burner supplements are believed to function by boosting your resting metabolic rate, with their active ingredients aiding in the reduction of body fat. The effectiveness of fat burner supplements remains uncertain. While they are widely used for weight loss, there is limited evidence to support their claims. These supplements often promise to block fat or carbohydrate absorption, suppress appetite, or boost metabolism. However, some may also interact with other medications you are taking. Fat burner supplements don't cause fat cells to vanish instantly. Instead, they support weight loss through various mechanisms, such as:

- Boosting your metabolism
- Decreasing the amount of fat your body absorbs
- Suppressing your appetite

What are the benefits of fat burners?

In order to dive into all the benefits of fat burners, we need to understand what some of the ingredients in fat burners are and what they do.

Guarana

Guarana, a plant native to the Amazon, is well-known for its caffeine-rich seeds and is commonly found in energy drinks, dietary supplements, and fat burners.

The primary fat-burning effect of guarana comes from its high caffeine content. As a stimulant for the central nervous system, caffeine can boost thermogenesis, leading to increased calorie burning. Guarana is also a key ingredient in products like Lipitek and The Burner, as well as some pre-workout formulas.

Benefits of Guarana:

- Enhances thermogenesis, promoting greater calorie burn.
- May boost athletic performance, energy levels, and mental focus.

Capsaicin

Capsaicin, the active compound responsible for the spiciness of red chilies, is widely used as a dietary supplement for weight loss due to its thermogenic and appetite-suppressing properties. But how does Capsaicin support weight loss?

Capsaicin can boost thermogenesis, helping to accelerate

metabolism and promote fat burning.

Capsaicin can also reduce your appetite. Research indicates that capsaicin may help reduce appetite, potentially leading to lower calorie intake.

Capsaicin offers a more organic approach to weight loss, making it an appealing option for those seeking natural solutions.

Carnitine

Carnitine is a molecule essential for transporting fatty acids into the mitochondria, where they are burned to generate energy. It is a key ingredient in lipotropic fat burners and is commonly found in L-carnitine supplements, as well as in carnitine-infused water and drinks.

Carnitine enhances endurance. It facilitates the use of fat as an energy source, supporting improved stamina. Carnitine also reduces fatigue which may aid in promoting better post-workout recovery.

Capsaicin can also reduce your appetite. Research indicates that capsaicin may help reduce appetite, potentially leading to lower calorie intake.

Capsaicin offers a more organic approach to weight loss, making it an appealing option for those seeking natural solutions.

What are the negatives of fat burners?

While fat burners can be helpful for some, they may also cause side effects depending on the ingredients and an individual's sensitivity. Common side effects include:

Increased Heart Rate: Thermogenic fat burners can elevate heart rate, which may be risky for individuals with heart conditions.

Insomnia: Stimulants like caffeine can disrupt sleep patterns, negatively impacting recovery and performance.

Gastrointestinal Issues: Some ingredients may cause stomach upset, nausea, or diarrhea.

Anxiety and Irritability: Stimulants can also affect mood, potentially increasing anxiety and irritability.

It's important to follow the recommended dosage for fat burners, as overdosing can significantly increase the risk of side effects.

Consumption

Always follow the recommended dosage provided on the label or as advised by a healthcare professional. Overuse can lead to side effects.

I recommended taking fat burners with a full glass of water to aid absorption and prevent stomach irritation.

Many fat burners are best taken in the morning or before workouts, especially those containing stimulants like caffeine, as they can boost energy and metabolism. If the fat burner contains stimulants, avoid taking it late in the day to prevent disrupting sleep.

Fat burners can be effective for weight loss and performance enhancement, but they may also lead to side effects. Understanding these potential risks can help you use these supplements more safely and effectively.

When used for extended periods, fat burners can lose their effectiveness as the body adapts. For this reason, it's recommended to take them in cycles, ideally for two to three months, especially at the beginning of a diet.

8

Conclusion

In this book, I reviewed several popular supplements, each serving a unique purpose for enhancing performance and supporting fitness goals. Here's a summary of the key points:

- **Protein powder** is a staple for many fitness enthusiasts, helping to meet protein needs, especially when whole food options are less convenient. Whey protein is one of the most popular forms due to its quick absorption, though plant-based options are available for those with dietary restrictions. Consuming protein post-workout aids muscle recovery and growth.

- **Creatine** is an effective supplement for improving strength, muscle mass, and performance. While it's highly beneficial, some individuals may experience water retention or digestive discomfort.

- **Pre-workout supplements** help boost energy, endurance, and focus during workouts. They can be effective, but be cautious with stimulants like caffeine to avoid jitteriness or digestive issues. It's always a good idea to start with smaller doses to assess your tolerance.

- **Amino acids**, especially **Essential Amino Acids (EAAs)** and **Branched-Chain Amino Acids (BCAAs)**, are crucial for muscle repair and growth. While BCAAs can be helpful, EAAs are a more comprehensive choice as they provide all the essential building blocks for muscle protein synthesis.

- **Mass gainers** are high-calorie supplements designed to help individuals struggling to gain weight or muscle. While they can be effective, they're not a miracle solution and may cause digestive discomfort. Whole food meals should be prioritized for long-term results.

- **Fat burners** are used for weight loss by boosting metabolism, suppressing appetite, and increasing fat burning. Ingredients like caffeine and capsaicin can offer some benefits, but fat burners come with risks, including side effects like increased heart rate, insomnia, and gastrointestinal issues.

Supplements, including protein powders, can support your fitness journey, but they should complement a solid foundation of whole foods, proper training, and adequate rest. Supplements aren't magic pills—consistency and dedication to your overall health are key. Protein powder, for instance, can help ensure you're getting enough protein to support muscle growth, but it shouldn't replace balanced meals.

Your path to fitness success is built on the choices you make every day. Keep focusing on what you can control, and trust that every effort you put in brings you closer to your goals. You're capable of achieving everything you set your mind to. Keep pushing, stay motivated, and don't forget to celebrate the small victories along the way!

If you found this book helpful, I'd love to hear your thoughts. Please consider leaving a review on Amazon.

If you need additional help you can find me on Instagram: https://www.instagram.com/alexander.filevski/

Thank you for reading this book and good luck!

Alexander

9

References:

Nordqvist, J. (2023, June 26). *Should I use creatine supplements?* https://www.medicalnewstoday.com/articles/263269#should_I_use_creatine_supplements

Cissn, R. M. M. (2023, November 2). *Everything you need to know about Creatine.* Healthline. https://www.healthline.com/nutrition/what-is-creatine#muscle-gain

Cissn, G. T. P. C. (2023, July 17). *Top 6 types of creatine reviewed.* Healthline. https://www.healthline.com/nutrition/types-of-creatine

Rd, J. K. M. (2023, August 7). *Essential amino acids: definition, benefits, and food sources.* Healthline.

Taylor, M. (2024, February 29). *What are fat burner supplements?* WebMD. https://www.webmd.com/vitamins-and-supplements/what-are-fat-burner-supplements

REFERENCES:

Cpt, E. L. M. R. (2021, December 13). *Should you take Pre-Workout supplements?* Healthline. https://www.healthline.com/nutrition/pre-workout-supplements#basics

Usaw-L, J. D. N., & Usaw-L, J. D. N. (2024, November 22). *Everything you need to know about mass gainers.* BarBend. https://barbend.com/mass-gainers/

Shaikh, J., MD. (2021, October 18). *Is it good to take mass gainers? side effects.* MedicineNet. https://www.medicinenet.com/is_it_good_to_take_mass_gainers/article.htm

WHEY PROTEIN: Overview, uses, side effects, precautions, interactions, dosing and reviews. (n.d.). https://www.webmd.com/vitamins/ai/ingredientmono-833/whey-protein

Rdn, V. A. (2024, October 24). *Protein powder: Everything you need to know.* culinahealth.com. https://culinahealth.com/everything-you-need-to-know-about-protein-powders/

Leonard, J. (2023, March 10). *What are the benefits of protein powder?* https://www.medicalnewstoday.com/articles/323093#takeaway

www.ingramcontent.com/pod-product-compliance
Lightning Source LLC
Chambersburg PA
CBHW051859250726
48659CB00006B/2305